ENTRY THREATS AND PRICING IN THE GENERIC DRUG INDUSTRY

Brett Wendling*
Steven Tenn

Federal Trade Commission

June 3, 2010

Abstract

We provide the first analysis of potential competition in the generic drug industry. Our identification strategy exploits a provision of the Hatch-Waxman Act that rewards 180 days of marketing exclusivity to the first generic drug applicant against the holder of a branded drug patent. This provision creates observable drug-level variation in both actual and potential competition that allows us to identify their separate effects. We find mixed evidence of price being used as a strategic entry deterrent. In smaller drug markets where entry is more easily deterred, we find that price falls in response to an increase in potential competition. We also find that few manufacturers enter these markets after the Hatch-Waxman exclusivity period, indicating this price reduction is an effective deterrent. In contrast, in larger drug markets the incumbent accommodates entry by lowering price only after competing manufacturers enter the market.

Keywords: potential competition, entry deterrence, pharmaceutical, pricing
JEL Classification Codes: L11, L13, L65

ENTRY THREATS AND PRICING IN THE GENERIC DRUG INDUSTRY

I.   Introduction

It is well recognized that an incumbent may deter potential competitors by taking strategic action that reduces the profitability of entry. However, the use of price as a strategic entry deterrent is controversial since it may be profitable for the incumbent to raise price after entry has occurred, making its commitment to a low, entry-deterring price incredible. Depending on the theoretical model used to explain the link between the incumbent's pre-entry price and an entrant's expected profits, the effect of potential competition can vary from being extremely strong to entirely ineffectual in constraining market power (Gilbert 1989a,b). This wide range of theoretical outcomes highlights the need for empirical analysis to determine the real-world importance of potential competition.

Ideally, one would measure the effect of exogenous changes in potential competition after controlling for other relevant industry factors. In practice, however, it has proved difficult to account for changes in potential competition since they are often unobservable. Consequently, empirical evidence of potential competition is far more limited than support for the impact of actual competition (see Section II).

We provide the first analysis of potential competition in the generic drug industry. Our identification strategy exploits the "Drug Price Competition and Patent Term Restoration Act of 1984," commonly known as the Hatch-Waxman Act. This regulation has several provisions that encourage generic entry into prescription drug markets. The provision relevant to our analysis gives generic drug firms incentive to challenge branded drug patents.[1] It allows a generic drug manufacturer to include a "paragraph IV certification" in its Abbreviated New Drug Application (ANDA) to the Food and Drug Administration (FDA) that its version of the drug will either not

---

[1] The more widely known provision of the Act replaces the original generic drug approval process with an Abbreviated New Drug Application. This regulatory change significantly increased generic entry (Berndt 2002).

infringe on the FDA's Orange Book patents, or that the relevant Orange Book patents are invalid.[2] The Hatch-Waxman Act encourages generic firms to incur litigation costs by rewarding 180 days of marketing exclusivity to the first to file an ANDA with a paragraph IV certification.[3] This marketing exclusivity period protects the designated first-filer from competition with other generic entrants.[4] Following the end of the exclusivity period, two changes occur. First, there may be variation in actual competition as other generic drug manufacturers enter the market. Second, regardless of whether entry occurs, there is the threat of (additional) entry that does not exist during the exclusivity period. Since the Hatch-Waxman Act creates observable variation in both actual and potential competition, we can separately identify their impact on price.

Our analysis of the effect of potential competition on price employs a treatment-control group framework.[5] The treatment group consists of generic drugs that received marketing exclusivity during the initial 180 days. We measure the change in price between the exclusivity period and the following period where the Hatch-Waxman Act does not prohibit entry. When measuring this price change we control for other factors that vary between the two periods, including the number of actual competitors. We compare this to a counterpart price change for drugs that were not granted an exclusivity period. The key difference between the two sets of drugs is that the former experiences a change in potential competition after the first 180 days,

---

[2] In these instances, the FDA may not approve the generic drug until 30 months after the generic files its drug application with the FDA or after a favorable decision in the patent litigation, if earlier.

[3] Prior to 2003, the first-to-file generic manufacturer could be distinguished by the exact minute a drug application was submitted. If several firms provided valid applications on the same day, the FDA would grant exclusivity to the first applicant. This provision has since been relaxed and now multiple firms can be designated as the first-filer.

[4] As noted in footnote 3, the FDA may designate multiple manufacturers as the first-filer. Note, however, that this will not lead to variation in the number of manufacturers within the exclusivity period since additional entry is prohibited by the Hatch-Waxman Act. The only exception is the Act does not stop the branded drug manufacturer from introducing an "authorized generic" during the exclusivity period. Authorized generics typically enter at the beginning of exclusivity, leading to little variation in competition within the period.

[5] Generic drugs are homogenous products with little differentiation across manufacturers. As such, entry deterrence is most likely to occur along the price dimension.

while the latter does not. Our "difference in difference" estimator uses this variation to capture the impact of potential competition on generic drug prices.

We find mixed evidence of price being used as a strategic entry deterrent in the generic drug industry. For small drug markets, where it is easier to deter entry due to lower expected profits, we find that price falls in response to an increase in potential competition. Few manufacturers enter these markets following expiration of the Hatch-Waxman exclusivity period, indicating this price reduction is an effective deterrent. In contrast, in larger drug markets where entry deterrence is less likely to be successful, the incumbent maintains a high price until forced to respond to actual competition.

The layout of the paper is as follows. Section II reviews the preceding literature. Section III details the dataset employed. Our identification approach is discussed in Section IV. Section V presents the econometric methodology and reports results. Section VI concludes.

II.   Literature Review

In early models of potential competition, the incumbent commits to sell the "limit quantity" (and charges the corresponding "limit price") where the residual demand faced by a potential entrant is insufficient to support profitable entry (Bain 1949, Modigliani 1958, Sylos-Labini 1962, Dixit 1979).[6] Factors that affect the feasibility of a limit-pricing strategy include fixed entry costs, returns to scale, and product differentiation. The key assumption in the limit-pricing framework is that the incumbent commits to sell the limit quantity regardless of whether entry actually occurs. This assumption has been criticized in the subsequent literature since, if entry occurs, the profit maximizing strategy for the incumbent may be to accommodate the

---

[6] See Gilbert (1989a,b) and Bergman (2003) for discussion of strategic entry deterrence via non-price mechanisms. For example, Spence (1977) and Dixit (1980) analyze investment in capacity.

entrant by reducing output. When this is recognized by a forward-looking potential entrant, limit pricing may not be a credible entry deterrent.[7]

One way of overcoming this weakness of the limit-pricing framework is to incorporate cost uncertainty into the model (Salop 1979, Milgrom and Roberts 1982). If an entrant cannot observe the incumbent's costs, the incumbent may deter entry by setting a low price to signal it is a low cost firm or to hide the fact it is a high cost firm.

An alternative approach to modeling the effect of potential competition is the "contestable markets" theory (Baumol et al. 1982). This framework relies on several strong assumptions that include zero sunk costs of entry and that an entrant can capture the entire market by undercutting the incumbent's price. In a contestable market, a monopolist incumbent is so constrained by potential competition that it cannot make positive profits. Otherwise, entry could profitably occur since the entrant is assumed to have the same costs as the incumbent.

The models described above provide avenues through which potential competition may affect incumbent pricing. However, each model provides a very different description of the nature of potential competition. Moreover, the models characterize conditions under which potential competition does not lead to lower prices. This wide range of theoretical outcomes highlights the need for empirical analysis to determine the importance of potential competition.

Relatively little empirical research examines the effects of potential competition. In their reviews of the literature, Gilbert (1989a,b) and Bergman (2003) discuss the problem of measuring potential competition and separately identifying its impact from correlated market factors that also affect price. Due to these difficulties, empirical research has largely focused on the airline industry, where institutional factors facilitate the measurement of potential competitors (Morrison and Winston 1987, Strassmann 1990, Kwoka 2001, Goolsbee and Syverson 2008). This research generally finds that the incumbent responds to potential entry by

---

[7] See also the literature on "dynamic limit pricing" (Gaskins 1971, Judd and Peterson 1986). A limitation of this group of models is that the link between the incumbent's price and the likelihood of future entry is exogenously specified or restricted in a particular way.

lowering price, but the impact of a potential entrant is less than the effect of a realized entrant. Of course, this finding may not apply to industries that face different competitive conditions.[8]

Empirical Pharmaceutical Literature

The prescription drug industry has been used extensively to evaluate the effect of entry on price. This is due to both the importance of the industry to the overall economy, and because the large number of independent, yet comparable, drug markets facilitates statistical analysis. Researchers generally find the impact of realized entry differs for branded and generic drugs (Caves et al. 1991, Graboski and Vernon 1992, Griliches and Cockburn 1994, Lu and Comanor 1998, Reiffen and Ward 2005, Regan 2008). While generic drug prices decline in the number of generic manufacturers, branded drug prices either increase or stay the same. A related literature finds that generic entry is more likely to occur in larger drug markets (Frank and Salkever 1997, Scott Morton 1999).

A smaller set of papers analyzes the impact of potential competition in the pharmaceutical industry. Ellison and Ellison (2007) develop a theory in which the incumbent's investment is non-monotonic with respect to market size when firms respond to potential entrants. They find support for non-monotonicity with respect to advertising and research and development in branded drug markets. They interpret this result as evidence of incumbent response to potential entry. Bergman and Rudholm (2003) analyze Swedish data and find that branded drug prices decline following an increase in potential competition due to patent expiration. Cool et al. (1999) exploits the New Drug Application (NDA) approval changes in the 1962 amendment to the "Food, Drugs, and Cosmetics Act," as well as the presence of firms in

---

[8] A few papers examine the effect of potential competition in other industries. For example, Savage and Wirth (2005) and Lee et al. (2006) consider the cable television and telecommunications industries, respectively. Below, we discuss papers that focus on prescription drugs.

different therapeutic classes, to identify the effects of potential competition on branded drugs.[9] They find that firm profitability is curbed by the threat of competition.

All of these papers analyze the impact of potential competition on branded drugs. To our knowledge, our study is the first to analyze the impact of potential competition on generic drug prices. As noted above, a large number of studies show that the effect of actual competition by generic manufacturers significantly differs for branded and generic drugs. This suggests that the literature's findings regarding potential competition in the branded drug industry may not apply to generic drugs. Consequently, it is important to analyze the effect of potential competition specifically in that industry.

III.   Data

Our analysis employs monthly wholesale data from IMS pharmaceutical services. This dataset reports sales for every oral solid prescription medication distributed in the United States over the period January 2003 to December 2008.[10] Sales are reported separately by drug, which is defined as a unique combination of molecule, dosage form, strength, and therapeutic class. The IMS data is combined with information from the FDA regarding when the Hatch-Waxman exclusivity period occurs for each drug (where applicable).

Data from the quarter prior to first generic entry is used to measure the market size of each drug, which is employed in our analysis. Due to this need for pre-entry data, we restrict the dataset to drugs that first faced generic competition after April 2003. We also exclude over-the-counter medications, vitamins and decongestants. These drugs are distributed in sales channels that IMS does not survey. In addition, they often change active ingredients over time, which

---

[9] The change required firms to provide evidence that a drug is both safe and efficacious. Prior to the enactment of this law, drug firms only had to demonstrate their product was safe.

[10] An "oral solid" is a drug sold in tablet or capsule form.

makes them difficult to track from year to year. These restrictions lead to a data sample of 312 drugs, of which 123 were granted a 180-day exclusivity period under the Hatch-Waxman Act.

A striking feature of the data is that dollar sales are highly skewed. The smallest drug in our sample represents less than a million dollars in annual sales while the largest drug has over $2.5 billion in sales, where market size is measured as annualized branded drug sales in the quarter prior to first generic entry. Market size is a key determinant of the number of entrants in drug markets (Frank and Salkever 1997, Scott Morton 1999). Consequently, in much of our analysis we split the sample by whether a drug's market size is above or below the median. Table 1 shows that, on average, there are 2.7 generic manufacturers in small drug markets compared to 5.8 manufacturers in large drug markets. We consider whether this difference in the number of generic entrants affects the feasibility of using price as a strategic entry deterrent.

We motivate our empirical analysis by comparing price trends for generic drugs with and without an exclusivity period. Following standard practice in the literature (Caves et al. 1991), we scale each generic price by the corresponding branded drug's pre-entry price to arrive at a price measure that can be compared across drugs. For each generic drug d in time t, we calculate $p_{dt} = p_{dt}^g / p_d^b$, where p_d^b and p_{dt}^g are branded and generic drug prices, respectively. Note that p_d^b does not have a time subscript since it corresponds to the branded drug's price in the quarter prior to generic entry. When calculating the generic drug price p_{dt}^g we aggregate across all generic manufacturers of a given drug, weighting by volume sales (i.e., price is calculated as total dollar sales across all generic manufacturers divided by total quantity).

Figure 1 presents the mean price ratio p_{dt} for drugs with and without a Hatch-Waxman exclusivity period. Drugs with an exclusivity period initially set a much higher price. During the Hatch-Waxman exclusivity period, drugs with exclusivity are approximately 30% more expensive, on average. This price difference persists for the full 6-month exclusivity period. After the Hatch-Waxman exclusivity period ends, the two price series start to converge and they are quite similar by month eight. These price trends are the result of changes in both actual and potential competition. Once the Hatch-Waxman exclusivity period ends, additional generic competitors enter the market and there is the threat of future entry. The goal of this study is to determine to what extent the price decline that follows the end of the exclusivity period is due to actual versus potential competition.

IV.   The Hatch-Waxman Act and Identification of Potential Competition

In this section, we describe in further detail how the Hatch-Waxman Act allows us to identify the effect of potential competition on generic drug pricing. Consider the following timeline of the first-filing generic manufacturer's incentive to engage in strategic entry deterrence for drugs that enter via a paragraph IV certification.

Hatch-Waxman Timeline

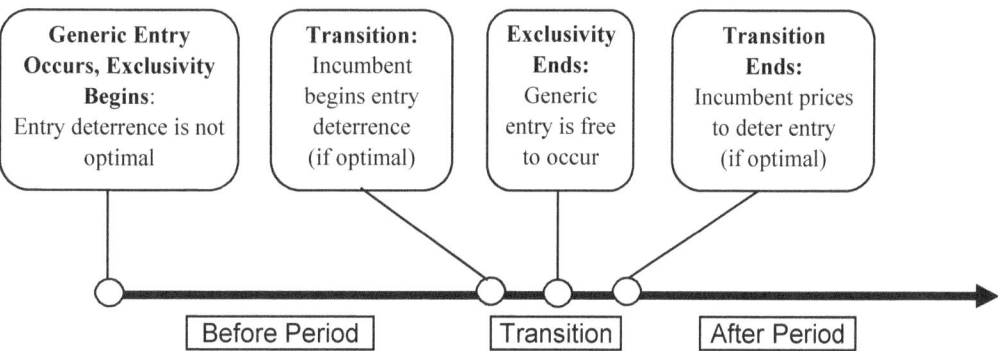

The Hatch-Waxman Act grants a 180-day exclusivity period to the first-filing generic drug applicant against a holder of a branded drug patent. There is little incentive for the first-filer to engage in entry deterrence at the beginning of the exclusivity period. Doing so would be a costly exercise without any offsetting benefit since entry by independent generic firms is prohibited by the Hatch-Waxman Act. After the exclusivity period ends, however, the incumbent firm may find entry deterrence to be a profitable strategy since entry is no longer restricted by the Act.

Although expiration of the exclusivity period clearly delineates when independent firms can enter the market, it is possible that firms initiate entry deterrence prior to the end of exclusivity. This may be the case, for example, if it takes time to implement a price change or if the incumbent wants to signal its pricing strategy to potential entrants. Similarly, the transition to an entry-deterring price may not be finished prior to expiration of the Hatch-Waxman exclusivity period. For these reasons, the pricing strategy during the transition period surrounding expiration of the exclusivity period is likely a mixture of the price strategies employed in the prior and subsequent periods.

An incumbent would like to defer an entry deterring price reduction in order to reap higher profits for as long as possible. Consequently, the transition period surrounding the end of the exclusivity period is likely to be relatively short. However, we are not aware of any institutional market features that provide guidance regarding its duration. Our analysis therefore explores several specifications for the transition period. We employ a 1-month transition window in the baseline model, but also consider a 2-month window as well as no transition period at all.

The analysis compares prices in the "before" period, which consists of the first part of the exclusivity period where entry deterrence is not optimal, to prices in the post-exclusivity "after" period that follows the transition to an entry deterring price (if optimal). Since the pricing strategy during the transition window is unclear, we do not use this period to identify the effect of potential competition. A price decline following expiration of the exclusivity period would be evidence that price is used as a strategic entry deterrent. However, our analysis recognizes that other factors may affect the change in price between these two periods. Most notably, entry may occur. In addition, the Hatch-Waxman exclusivity period is potentially correlated with life-cycle effects that affect drug pricing. To account for these factors we employ a "difference in difference" estimator that compares the change in price for drugs that have an exclusivity period to the price change for drugs that do not.

Specifically, we estimate the effect of potential competition on generic drug prices using a commonly employed two-stage method (Donald and Lang 2007). In the first stage, we calculate each drug's price change after the exclusivity period, or after the first 6 months following initial generic entry for drugs without an exclusivity period. When calculating these price changes we control for other factors that affect price, including changes in actual competition. In the second stage, we test whether the price change for drugs granted an exclusivity period under the Hatch-Waxman Act differs from the price change for non-exclusive drugs. Since the key difference between the two sets of drugs is that one experiences a change in potential competition upon completion of the Hatch-Waxman exclusivity period, while the other does not, our difference in difference estimator measures the effect of potential competition on generic drug prices.

This approach of using a control group, and including additional controls to account for any differences between the two groups, has been widely applied in prior research.[11] Our estimation strategy is closely related to the method used by Bergman and Rudholm (2003) to measure the effect of potential competition on branded drug prices. Bergman and Rudholm use the expiration of the branded drug's patent as a source of variation in potential competition in the same manner we exploit the expiration of the Hatch-Waxman exclusivity period.

A key benefit of the Hatch-Waxman Act is that it provides an exogenous source of variation in potential competition since the Act was written decades prior to the entry events studied in this paper. A second advantage of our study is that we analyze the effect of the Hatch-Waxman Act across a large number of drug markets. Our focus on numerous, independent events that occur at different points in time provides a robust source of variation in potential competition. In addition, the diverse timing of these events allows us to control for calendar time and product life-cycle effects in a flexible manner.

V.   Empirical Analysis

Our difference in difference estimator is implemented in two stages. In the first stage, we estimate equation (1) to obtain each drug's change in price between the exclusivity and non-

_____

[11] See Bertrand et al. (2004) and the citations contained therein for discussion of the "difference in difference" estimation approach. Bertrand et al. recommend the two-stage estimation strategy that we employ.

exclusivity periods after controlling for a set of variables X_{dt} that includes the number of competitors in the market as well as other factors (as discussed below).

(1) $\quad \ln p_{dt}^g = \phi_d + \phi_t + \delta_d^0 PRE_{dt} + \delta_d^1 TRANS_{dt} + \delta_d^2 POST_{dt} + X_{dt}\beta + \varepsilon_{dt}$

Dependent variable $\ln p_{dt}^g$ is the log price of generic drug d in month t. Variables ϕ_d and ϕ_t are drug and time fixed effects, respectively. PRE_{dt}, $TRANS_{dt}$, and $POST_{dt}$ are dummy variables for three mutually exclusive periods corresponding to the "before," "transition," and "after" event windows. Note that coefficients $\{\delta_d^0, \delta_d^1, \delta_d^2\}$ for these variables have a drug d subscript indicating a separate effect is estimated for each drug (i.e., we interact PRE_{dt}, $TRANS_{dt}$, and $POST_{dt}$ with a set of drug fixed effects).

We treat a month as being part of the exclusivity period if the end of marketing exclusivity occurs on the 28th day of the month or later. That is, a month is treated as occurring during the exclusivity period only if it is almost entirely composed of exclusive days, with at most three non-exclusive days. The "before" window is defined to correspond to the Hatch-Waxman exclusivity period, or the first 6 months after initial generic entry for drugs without an exclusivity period. The "transition" period is the single month following the before period, which generally contains a mixture of exclusive and non-exclusive days (for drugs with an exclusivity period).[12] The "after" window is the following 12 months.[13]

Equation (1) contains additional variables X_{dt} that control for changes occurring between the before and after periods. This set includes fixed effects for the number of months elapsed since first generic entry. In addition, we control for changes in actual competition by including a set of dummy variables for the number of generic manufacturers.[14] For small drugs, sales sometimes occur irregularly; one or two months without sales can represent standard

---

[12] Later in this section, we consider alternative definitions for the transition period.

[13] The period following the after window is the omitted time category.

[14] When counting the number of manufacturers we exclude drug repackagers.

business practice rather than exit. We assume a manufacturer has exited a particular drug market only after four consecutive months of zero sales.[15] Authorized generics are included in the count of manufacturers.[16] To account for the possibility that the competitive effect of an authorized generic differs from the impact of an independent generic manufacturer (Reiffen and Ward 2007, Federal Trade Commission 2009), we include an indicator for the presence of an authorized generic and interact this variable with the number of generic manufacturers and its square.

Estimates from equation (1) are used to calculate $\Delta \ln p_d = \delta_d^2 - \delta_d^0$, the change in log price between the before and after windows after controlling for the number of generic manufacturers and the other variables contained in X_{dt}. This measure is the dependent variable in the second stage of the analysis.[17]

$$(2) \qquad \Delta \ln p_d = \alpha EXCL_d + Z_d \gamma + \mu_d$$

Variable $EXCL_d$ is an indicator for whether drug d had an exclusivity period. The model also controls for additional drug characteristics Z_d that potentially explain the change in price between the event windows. This set of additional controls includes an indicator for whether the drug has an authorized generic, the drug's market size percentile, a set of dummy variables for dosage form (tablet, capsule, etc.), and a set of fixed effects for therapeutic class.[18]

The key variable of interest in equation (2) is coefficient α on the exclusivity variable $EXCL_d$. This effect is our "difference in difference" estimator, and measures the change in

---

[15] The date of exit is backdated to the period following the last observed sale. For example, if a manufacturer has positive sales in month 4, but zero sales in months 5-8, then that manufacturer is considered to have exited between month 4 and 5.

[16] An "authorized generic" is a drug approved by the FDA as a branded drug, but marketed as a generic.

[17] In equation 2, each observation corresponds to a particular drug (in contrast, in equation 1 an observation is a drug-month combination). It is not possible to calculate $\Delta \ln p_d$ for 31 drugs where first generic entry occurs in the last 7 months of the data (June 2008 or later), since the after period is never observed. The second stage regression includes 281 drugs from the full sample of 312.

[18] Therapeutic classes with fewer than five drugs in a given regression are grouped together into an "other" category. As before, market size is measured as the corresponding branded drug's annualized sales in the quarter prior to first generic entry.

price between the before and after periods for drugs with exclusivity relative to a control group of non-exclusive drugs. The key identification assumption is that non-exclusive drugs are a valid control group for drugs with an exclusivity period after controlling for variables X_{dt} and Z_d in equations (1) and (2). Any remaining difference between the two sets of drugs is assumed to be due to potential competition; drugs with an exclusivity period face an increase in potential competition after the period ends, which does not occur for their non-exclusive counterparts. Our difference in difference estimator captures this change, allowing us to measure the effect of an increase in potential competition on generic drug prices. We use all non-exclusive drugs as the control group in the baseline model. As a robustness check, later in this section we consider an alternative control group consisting of drugs that submitted a paragraph IV certification but did not receive an exclusivity period.

Table 2 presents the first and second stage regression estimates. Robust standard errors are reported that cluster by molecule. This accounts for any correlation in unobserved characteristics across drugs with the same active ingredient. The first stage results demonstrate the importance of controlling for realized competition. Consistent with prior research, we find that additional competitors lead to lower prices. However, some of the individual coefficients are imprecisely estimated and are not always statistically significant at conventional levels. Competitor type also matters. Generic drug prices are higher when one of the competing manufacturers is an authorized generic, although this effect decreases in the number of competitors.[19]

In the second stage results, the key effect of interest is the coefficient for whether a drug had an exclusivity period, which is our difference in difference estimator. The price of exclusive

---

[19] While the coefficient estimate for the authorized generic dummy may appear to suggest that prices are considerably higher in markets with an authorized generic, the interactions between the authorized generic dummy and the number of manufacturers dampen this effect. In the average market with 4.2 manufacturers, the net impact on price of an authorized generic, holding the total number of manufacturers constant, is 13.8% (SE=8.1%), which is not statistically significant at the 5% level. The net impact of an authorized generic is statistically significant only when there are three or fewer manufacturers (including the authorized generic).

drugs falls by 11.8% (SE=8.4%) after the exclusivity period ends, relative to the price change for non-exclusive drugs. However, this effect is not statistically significant at any conventional level.

A key determinant of whether a firm engages in strategic entry deterrence is the cost of deterring potential competitors. It is likely that entry deterrence is costlier in large markets, due to their greater profitability. Consequently, an entry-deterring pricing strategy may not be profit maximizing in these markets. To test this hypothesis we split the sample by market size. Drugs with market size above and below the median are referred to as "large" and "small" markets, respectively.

Table 3 reports results from estimating the model separately for small and large drug markets. The effect of the exclusivity period is very different for the two sets of drugs. In small drug markets, the price of exclusive drugs falls by 19.4% (SE=9.2%) relative to non-exclusive drugs. This effect is statistically significant at the 5% level. In contrast, in larger drug markets price does not change in response to potential competition. This finding is consistent with the hypothesis that it is not profitable to deter entry in larger markets where entry is highly likely to occur. Instead, the incumbent generic manufacturer reduces price only when forced to respond to actual entry.

These results suggest that price is used as an entry deterrent in small drug markets, but not in large drug markets. We now explore whether price is an *effective* entry deterrent by estimating equations (1) and (2) using the log number of manufacturers as the dependent variable, rather than price.[20] If price is an effective entry deterrent in small drug markets, one should see relatively little entry following the end of the exclusivity period. Similarly, if firms accommodate entry in large drug markets then entry should be observed following the end of exclusivity in those markets.

_____

[20] Of course, controls for the number of manufacturers are omitted from the model.

The results from this analysis, reported in Table 4, are consistent with price being used as an entry deterrent in small but not large drug markets. Substantial entry is observed in large drug markets, with a 43.2% (SE=16.2%) increase in the number of manufacturers, relative to the change for non-exclusive drugs. In contrast, only a 15.4% (SE=13.4%) change is found in small drug markets, which is not statistically significant at any conventional level. For smaller drugs we cannot reject the hypothesis that the price reduction following an increase in potential competition is an effective entry deterrent.

Sensitivity Analysis

Recall that in our baseline specification we use a 1-month transition period and a 12-month after period. We now examine the robustness of our results to alternative definitions for these event windows. Specifically, we consider using 0, 1, and 2 transition months, and after windows of 6, 12, and 24 months.

The results of these robustness checks are reported in the first column of Table 5. As before, we find that for small drugs price falls in response to potential competition. The estimated price decline ranges from 15% to 22%, depending on the specification. The only instance where the effect of potential competition is not statistically significant at the 5% level is when a 2-month transition window is used in conjunction with a 6-month after window. Nonetheless, this effect is nearly statistically significant with a p-value of .051. As before, little price change is apparent in large drug markets. The point estimates are generally small in magnitude and are never statistically significant at any conventional level.

In the baseline model, we employ a control group consisting of all non-exclusive drugs. A potential problem is that manufacturers do not randomly decide which drugs should undergo a paragraph IV certification. Patent litigation is costly, and is more likely to be profitable when the expected return from a successful patent challenge is higher. As such, exclusive drugs tend to have a larger market size than non-exclusive drugs. Our analysis accounts for this difference by explicitly controlling for market size. Nonetheless, we recognize the possibility that unobservable differences between the treatment and control groups may remain, potentially biasing our results.

We now consider an alternative control group that consists of non-exclusive drugs that filed a paragraph IV certification but did not have a Hatch-Waxman exclusivity period. This occurs when the first-to-file generic firm loses the patent litigation, or reaches a settlement with the branded manufacturer prior to entry.[21] These non-exclusive drugs are more similar to exclusive drugs since both had a paragraph IV certification. Evidence of this is seen in the market size of the two sets of drugs; we could not reject, at any conventional level, the hypothesis that exclusive drugs have the same average market size as non-exclusive paragraph IV drugs.[22] The endogeneity of which drugs are certified under paragraph IV does not pose a problem to the analysis when this alternative control group is employed since both the treatment and control groups undergo the same selection process. The drawback of this alternative control group is that it is substantially smaller, leading to less precise results.[23]

The second column of results in Table 5 repeats the analysis after restricting the dataset to drugs with a paragraph IV certification. For small drug markets, the alternative control group leads to stronger results. The estimated price decline ranges from 22% to 29%, depending on the specification. Each estimate is statistically significant at the 5% level. As before, we do not find a statistically significant effect in large drug markets.

Table 6 reports the results of similar robustness checks using the log number of manufacturers as the dependent variable. Qualitatively similar, but less precise, estimates are again obtained. The difference with our earlier set of results is that the change in the number of

---

[21] Patent settlements involving paragraph IV drugs are generally agreements on when the first-filing generic firm may enter the market. The settlements do not involve post-entry activity such as pricing. See Federal Trade Commission (2010) for details.

[22] In contrast, when the control group consists of all non-exclusive drugs the difference in means is statistically significant at the 1% level.

[23] Restricting the data to drugs with a paragraph IV certification leads to a sample of 195 drugs.

manufacturers in large drug markets is not statistically significant in one specification. However, it is almost significant at the 5% level with a p-value of .051. Generally, the results using the paragraph IV drugs confirm the findings from our baseline specification. In small markets, where entry deterrent pricing is observed, there is little change in the number of competitors. We cannot reject the hypothesis that price is an effective entry deterrent in these markets. In contrast, in large drug markets where entry deterrence is not observed, the number of manufacturers increases after the exclusivity period expires.

As a final robustness check, we undertake the following falsification test. Rather than comparing the price change between the before and after periods, we compute the price change between the after period and a "post-after" window corresponding to the following 12 months. We estimate the same model as before, but now include a post-after indicator variable for each drug. For both exclusive and non-exclusive drugs, there is no change in potential competition between these two periods since the after and post-after windows both follow expiration of the Hatch-Waxman exclusivity period. If the control group is valid then this test should not reveal a significant difference between the treatment and control groups.

The results from this analysis are generally supportive of our two control groups (non-exclusive drugs and non-exclusive paragraph IV drugs).[24] In the log price regressions, we do not find a statistically significant difference between the treatment and control groups. For smaller drug markets, this is also the case for the log manufacturer regressions. The falsification test "fails" only for large drug markets when all non-exclusive drugs are employed as the control group.[25] The difference in difference estimate for this specification equals 18.1% (SE=7.8%), indicating that exclusive drugs have significantly more entry between the after and post-after

[24] We conduct the falsification test using the baseline model employed earlier in this section that has a 1-month transition and a 12-month after period. On average, we observe 34 months of data for each drug. It is not practical to use a 24-month after window since relatively few drugs would have much post-after data, since that period starts in month 32 (6 month before window plus a 1 month transition plus a 24 month after window). Use of a 2-month transition window or no transition at all leads to similar results.

[25] The test "passes" when non-exclusive paragraph IV drugs are the controls.

windows than their non-exclusive counterparts. This suggests that it takes more than 12 months for entrants to respond fully to the expiration of the exclusivity period. Apart from this exception, however, the results from the falsification test are consistent with our control groups being valid.

VI.   Conclusion

The importance of potential competition in constraining market power has long been recognized as a theoretical matter. However, empirical evidence regarding the effects of potential competition is relatively limited despite its importance in understanding the strategic behavior of firms. We add to the empirical literature by providing the first analysis of potential competition in the generic drug industry. This industry offers a large number of independent, yet comparable, drug markets that facilitate statistical analysis. Our identification strategy uses the Hatch-Waxman 180-day exclusivity period granted to the first generic drug applicant against a holder of a branded drug patent as an exogenous source of variation in potential competition that varies over time and across drugs.

Our analysis finds that the incumbent in smaller drug markets lowers price in response to an increase in potential competition, and this price reduction appears to be an effective entry deterrent. In larger drug markets, the incumbent accommodates entry by lowering price only after competing manufacturers enter the market. This pricing strategy leads to a significant increase in the number of competitors once the Hatch-Waxman exclusivity period ends. Overall, the results suggest that price can be an effective entry deterrent in certain circumstances where the cost of deterring entry is not too high.

References

Bain, Joe S. 1949. "A Note on Pricing in Monopoly and Oligopoly," *American Economic Review* 39(2): 448-64.

Baumol, William J., John C. Panzar, and Robert D. Willig. 1982. *Contestable Markets and the Theory of Industry Structure*. New York: Harcourt, Brace, Jovanovich.

Bergman, Mats A. 2003. "Potential Competition: Theory, Empirical Evidence, and Legal Practice," Working Paper, Swedish Competition Authority.

Bergman, Mats A. and Niklas Rudholm. 2003. "The Relative Importance of Actual and Potential Competition: Empirical Evidence from the Pharmaceuticals Market," *Journal of Industrial Economics* 51(4):455-67.

Berndt, Ernst R. 2002. "Pharmaceuticals in U.S. Health Care: Determinants of Quantity and Price," *Journal of Economic Perspectives* 16(4):45-66.

Bertrand, Marianne, Esther Duflo, and Sendhil Mullainathan. 2004. "How Much Should We Trust Differences-in-Differences Estimates?" *Quarterly Journal of Economics* 119(1):249-75.

Caves, Richard E., Michael D. Whinston, and Mark A. Hurwitz. 1991. "Patent Expiration, Entry, and Competition in the U.S. Pharmaceutical Industry," *Brookings Papers on Economic Activity. Microeconomics* 1-66.

Cool, Karel, Lars-Hendrik Roller, and Benoit Leleux. 1999. "The Relative Impact of Actual and Potential Rivalry on Firm Profitability in the Pharmaceutical Industry," *Strategic Management Journal* 20(1):1-14.

Dixit, Avinash. 1979. "A Model of Duopoly Suggesting a Theory of Entry Barriers," *Bell Journal of Economics* 10(1):20-32.

Dixit, Avinash. 1980. "The Role of Investment in Entry-Deterrence," *Economic Journal* 90(357):95-106.

Donald, Stephen G., and Kevin Lang. 2007. "Inference with Difference-in-Differences and Other Panel Data," *Review of Economics and Statistics* 89(2): 221-33.

Ellison, Glenn and Sara Fisher Ellison. 2007. "Strategic Entry Deterrence and the Behavior of Pharmaceutical Incumbents Prior to Patent Expiration," NBER Working Paper 13069.

Federal Trade Commission. 2009. *Authorized Generics: An Interim Report.* Available at: http://www.ftc.gov/os/2009/06/P062105authorizedgenericsreport.pdf

Federal Trade Commission Staff Report. 2010. *Pay-for-Delay: How Drug Company Pay-Offs Cost Consumers Billions.* Available at: http://www.ftc.gov/os/2010/01/100112payfordelayrpt.pdf

Frank, Richard G. and David S. Salkever. 1997. "Generic Entry and the Pricing of Pharmaceuticals," *Journal of Economics and Management Strategy* 6(1):75-90.

Gaskins, Darius W. 1971. "Dynamic Limit Pricing: Optimal Pricing under Threat of Entry," *Journal of Economic Theory* 3(3):306-22.

Gilbert, Richard J. 1989a. "The Role of Potential Competition in Industrial Organization," *Journal of Economic Perspectives* 3(3):107-27.

Gilbert, Richard J. 1989b. "Mobility Barriers and the Value of Incumbency," in *Handbook of Industrial Organization,* vol. 1, Richard Schmalensee and Robert Willig, eds. New York: North Holland.

Goolsbee, Austan and Chad Syverson. 2008. "How Do Incumbents Respond to the Threat of Entry? Evidence from the Major Airlines," *Quarterly Journal of Economics* 123(4):1611-33.

Grabowski, Henry G. and John M. Vernon. 1992. "Brand Loyalty, Entry, and Price Competition in Pharmaceuticals after the 1984 Drug Act," *Journal of Law and Economics* 35(2):331-50.

Griliches, Zvi and Ian Cockburn. 1994. "Generics and New Goods in Pharmaceutical Price Indexes," *American Economic Review* 84(5):1213-32.

Judd, Kenneth L and Bruce C. Petersen. 1986. "Dynamic Limit Pricing and Internal Finance," *Journal of Economic Theory* 39(2):368-99.

Kwoka, John E. 2001. "Non-Incumbent Competition: Mergers Involving Constraining and Prospective Competitors," *Case Western Law Review* 52:173-209.

Lee, Jongsu, Yeonbae Kim, Jeong-Dong Lee, and Yuri Park. 2006. "Estimating the Extent of Potential Competition in the Korean Mobile Telecommunications Market: Switching Costs and Number Portability," *International Journal of Industrial Organization* 24(1):107-24.

Lu, Z. John and William S. Comanor. 1998. "Strategic Pricing of New Pharmaceuticals," *Review of Economics and Statistics* 80(1):108-18.

Milgrom, Paul and John Roberts. 1982. "Limit Pricing and Entry under Incomplete Information: An Equilibrium Analysis," *Econometrica* 50(2):443-59.

Modigliani, Franco. 1958. "New Developments on the Oligopoly Front," *Journal of Political Economy* 66(3):215-32.

Morrison, Steven A. and Clifford Winston. 1987. "Empirical Implications and Tests of the Contestability Hypothesis," *Journal of Law and Economics* 30(1):53-66.

Regan, Tracy L. 2008. "Generic Entry, Price Competition, and Market Segmentation in the Prescription Drug Market," *International Journal of Industrial Organization* 26(4):930-48.

Reiffen, David and Michael R. Ward. 2005. "Generic Drug Industry Dynamics," *Review of Economics and Statistics* 87(1):37-49.

Reiffen, David and Michael R. Ward. 2007. "'Branded Generics' as a Strategy to Limit Cannibalization of Pharmaceutical Markets," *Managerial and Decision Economics* 28(4/5):251-65.

Salop, Steven C. 1979. "Strategic Entry Deterrence," *American Economic Review* 69(2):335-38.

Savage, Scott J. and Michael Wirth. 2005. "Price, Programming and Potential Competition in US Cable Television Markets," *Journal of Regulatory Economics* 27(1):25-46.

Scott Morton, Fiona M. 1999. "Entry Decisions in the Generic Pharmaceutical Industry," *RAND Journal of Economics* 30(3):421-40.

Spence, A. Michael. 1977. "Entry, Capacity, Investment and Oligopolistic Pricing," *Bell Journal of Economics* 8(2):534-44.

Strassmann, Diana L. 1990. "Potential Competition in the Deregulated Airlines," *Review of Economics and Statistics* 72(4):696-702.

Sylos-Labini, Paolo. 1962. *Oligopoly and Technical Progress*. Cambridge: Harvard University Press.

Table 1:
Summary Statistics

	(i) All Drug Markets		(ii) Small Drug Markets		(iii) Large Drug Markets	
	Mean	Std Dev	Mean	Std Dev	Mean	Std Dev
Fixed Characteristics:						
Had an Exclusivity Period	0.39	0.49	0.25	0.43	0.54	0.50
Had an Authorized Generic	0.49	0.50	0.29	0.46	0.68	0.47
Tablet	0.68	0.47	0.68	0.47	0.68	0.47
Capsule	0.12	0.32	0.13	0.34	0.10	0.30
Extended Release Tablet	0.13	0.33	0.10	0.30	0.15	0.36
Extended Release Capsule	0.04	0.18	0.04	0.19	0.03	0.18
Other Dosage Form	0.04	0.21	0.06	0.23	0.03	0.18
Time-varying Characteristics:						
Generic Price, Relative to Branded						
Drug Pre-Entry Price	0.47	0.30	0.57	0.27	0.37	0.28
Months Since First Generic Entry	22.86	16.43	23.02	16.31	22.69	16.54
Number of Generic Manufacturers	4.2	3.4	2.7	2.0	5.8	3.8
Number of Drugs	312		156		156	
Number of Drug-Months	10,787		5,545		5,242	

Notes: IMS wholesale price data, April 2003 to December 2008. Branded drug price is measured in the quarter prior to first generic entry. Market size is measured as annualized branded drug sales in the quarter prior to first generic entry. Drugs with market size above (below) the median are defined as large (small) markets.

Table 2:
Effect of the Hatch-Waxman Exclusivity Period on Generic Drug Prices

Stage 1 Regression
Dep Variable: Log Price

	Est	SE	
Authorized Generic (AG) Present	0.514	0.176	*
AG × # Manufacturers	-0.109	0.055	*
AG × # Manufacturers Squared	0.005	0.003	
Manufacturers = 2	-0.091	0.035	*
Manufacturers = 3	-0.087	0.056	
Manufacturers = 4	-0.109	0.065	
Manufacturers = 5	-0.221	0.077	*
Manufacturers = 6	-0.295	0.082	*
Manufacturers = 7	-0.362	0.108	*
Manufacturers = 8	-0.406	0.126	*
Manufacturers = 9	-0.455	0.152	*
Manufacturers = 10	-0.581	0.173	*
Manufacturers > 10	-0.819	0.246	*

Stage 2 Regression
Dep Variable: Change in Log Price After Exclusivity Ends

	Est	SE	
Had an Exclusivity Period	-0.118	0.084	
Had an Authorized Generic	0.039	0.087	
Market Size Percentile	-0.581	0.131	*
Capsule	-0.106	0.146	
Extended Release Tablet	0.168	0.060	*
Extended Release Capsule	0.006	0.089	
Other Dosage Form	-0.237	0.152	

Notes: Robust standard errors are reported that cluster by molecule. Statistical significance: *=5%.

Stage 1 Notes: The model also includes a set of drug fixed effects, time fixed effects, and a set of fixed effects for the number of months elapsed since first generic entry. In addition, for each drug it includes dummy variables for the before, transition, and after event windows. N=10,787 drug-months, R^2=.98, RMSE=.21.

Stage 2 Notes: The model also includes a set of fixed effects for therapeutic class. The dependent variable is estimated from the first stage regression. N=281 drugs, R^2=.47, RMSE=.33.

Table 3:
Effect of the Hatch-Waxman Exclusivity Period on Generic Drug Prices, Separately by Small and Large Drug Markets

Stage 1 Regression
Dep Variable: Log Price

	Small Drug Markets		Large Drug Markets	
	Est	SE	Est	SE
Authorized Generic (AG) Present	0.185	0.099	0.733	0.258 *
AG × # Manufacturers	-0.023	0.053	-0.174	0.061 *
AG × # Manufacturers Squared	0.006	0.005	0.008	0.003 *
Manufacturers = 2	-0.038	0.026	-0.181	0.117
Manufacturers = 3	-0.046	0.050	-0.183	0.107
Manufacturers = 4	-0.099	0.079	-0.198	0.098 *
Manufacturers = 5	-0.195	0.094 *	-0.332	0.095 *
Manufacturers = 6	-0.387	0.102 *	-0.300	0.102 *
Manufacturers = 7	-0.479	0.138 *	-0.351	0.128 *
Manufacturers = 8	-0.598	0.175 *	-0.381	0.144 *
Manufacturers = 9	-0.614	0.189 *	-0.424	0.154 *
Manufacturers = 10	-0.612	0.182 *	-0.536	0.176 *
Manufacturers > 10	-0.754	0.252 *	-0.799	0.227 *

Stage 2 Regression
Dep Variable: Change in Log Price After Exclusivity Ends

	Small Drug Markets		Large Drug Markets	
	Est	SE	Est	SE
Had an Exclusivity Period	-0.194	0.092 *	0.000	0.108
Had an Authorized Generic	-0.066	0.070	0.065	0.138
Market Size Percentile	-0.374	0.202	-0.752	0.307 *
Capsule	-0.123	0.128	-0.126	0.215
Extended Release Tablet	-0.012	0.054	0.278	0.095 *
Extended Release Capsule	0.011	0.065	-0.014	0.094
Other Dosage Form	-0.114	0.111	-0.165	0.363

Notes: Robust standard errors are reported that cluster by molecule. Statistical significance: *=5%.

Stage 1 Notes: The model also includes a set of drug fixed effects, time fixed effects, and a set of fixed effects for the number of months elapsed since first generic entry. In addition, for each drug it includes dummy variables for the before, transition, and after event windows. Small drug markets: N=5,545 drug-months, R^2=.99, RMSE=.12. Large drug markets: N=5,242 drug-months, R^2=.98, RMSE=.27.

Stage 2 Notes: The model also includes a set of fixed effects for therapeutic class. The dependent variable is estimated from the first stage regression. Small drug markets: N=141 drugs, R^2=.30, RMSE=.26. Large drug markets: N=140 drugs, R^2=.41, RMSE=.40.

Table 4:
Effect of the Hatch-Waxman Exclusivity Period on Number of Generic Manufacturers, Separately by Small and Large Drug Markets

Stage 2 Regression
Dep Variable: Change in Log Manufacturers After Exclusivity Ends

	Small Drug Markets		Large Drug Markets	
	Est	SE	Est	SE
Had an Exclusivity Period	0.154	0.134	0.432	0.162 *
Market Size Percentile	0.544	0.242 *	0.968	0.381 *
Capsule	0.083	0.134	0.181	0.334
Extended Release Tablet	0.265	0.213	-0.251	0.122 *
Extended Release Capsule	-0.072	0.158	-0.029	0.186
Other Dosage Form	-0.215	0.190	-0.368	0.145 *

Notes: Robust standard errors are reported that cluster by molecule. Statistical significance: *=5%.

Stage 1 Notes: The model includes a set of drug fixed effects, time fixed effects, and a set of fixed effects for the number of months elapsed since first generic entry. In addition, for each drug it includes dummy variables for the before, transition, and after event windows. Small drug markets: N=5,545 drug-months, R^2=.96, RMSE=.21. Large drug markets: N=5,242 drug-months, R^2=.99, RMSE=.22.

Stage 2 Notes: The model also includes a set of fixed effects for therapeutic class. The dependent variable is estimated from the first stage regression. Small drug markets: N=141 drugs, R^2=.17, RMSE=.39. Large drug markets: N=140 drugs, R^2=.42, RMSE=.50.

Table 5:
Effect of the Hatch-Waxman Exclusivity Period on Generic Drug Prices, Alternative Event Windows and Control Groups

		Control Group 1: All Non-Exclusive Drugs				Control Group 2: Non-Exclusive Paragraph IV Drugs			
Transition Period	After Period	Small Drug Markets		Large Drug Markets		Small Drug Markets		Large Drug Markets	
		Est	SE	Est	SE	Est	SE	Est	SE
None	6 months	-0.147	0.068 *	0.002	0.079	-0.215	0.096 *	-0.108	0.103
None	12 months	-0.168	0.076 *	0.021	0.088	-0.239	0.096 *	-0.079	0.108
None	24 months	-0.197	0.082 *	0.059	0.098	-0.265	0.103 *	-0.010	0.123
1 month	6 months	-0.169	0.082 *	-0.033	0.097	-0.265	0.114 *	-0.160	0.131
1 month	12 months	-0.194	0.092 *	0.000	0.108	-0.275	0.120 *	-0.127	0.127
1 month	24 months	-0.218	0.096 *	0.046	0.118	-0.294	0.129 *	-0.029	0.141
2 months	6 months	-0.176	0.089	-0.040	0.116	-0.272	0.109 *	-0.175	0.149
2 months	12 months	-0.203	0.100 *	-0.022	0.124	-0.260	0.117 *	-0.150	0.152
2 months	24 months	-0.217	0.102 *	0.035	0.136	-0.259	0.124 *	-0.049	0.175

Notes: Robust standard errors are reported that cluster by molecule. Statistical significance: *=5%. Each estimate corresponds to the coefficient for the "Had an Exclusivity Period" variable from the stage 2 regression. The model with a transition period of 1 month, an after period of 12 months, and using control group 1 corresponds to the baseline specification reported in Table 3.

Table 6:
Effect of the Hatch-Waxman Exclusivity Period on Number of Manufacturers,
Alternative Event Windows and Control Groups

| Transition Period | After Period | Control Group 1: All Non-Exclusive Drugs | | | | Control Group 2: Non-Exclusive Paragraph IV Drugs | | | |
| | | Small Drug Markets | | Large Drug Markets | | Small Drug Markets | | Large Drug Markets | |
		Est	SE	Est	SE	Est	SE	Est	SE
None	6 months	0.180	0.118	0.386	0.126 *	-0.050	0.199	0.404	0.130 *
None	12 months	0.150	0.126	0.406	0.147 *	-0.050	0.201	0.395	0.160 *
None	24 months	0.160	0.119	0.486	0.160 *	-0.026	0.197	0.454	0.185 *
1 month	6 months	0.196	0.129	0.429	0.136 *	-0.080	0.224	0.434	0.145 *
1 month	12 months	0.154	0.134	0.432	0.162 *	-0.051	0.224	0.411	0.183 *
1 month	24 months	0.169	0.124	0.515	0.171 *	-0.021	0.219	0.473	0.204 *
2 months	6 months	0.171	0.134	0.493	0.171 *	-0.141	0.255	0.498	0.200 *
2 months	12 months	0.125	0.137	0.501	0.195 *	-0.098	0.252	0.481	0.238
2 months	24 months	0.146	0.126	0.595	0.202 *	-0.088	0.245	0.562	0.268 *

Notes: Robust standard errors are reported that cluster by molecule. Statistical significance: *=5%. Each estimate corresponds to the coefficient for the "Had an Exclusivity Period" variable from the stage 2 regression. The model with a transition period of 1 month, an after period of 12 months, and using control group 1 corresponds to the baseline specification reported in Table 4.

Figure 1:
Average Price by Exclusivity

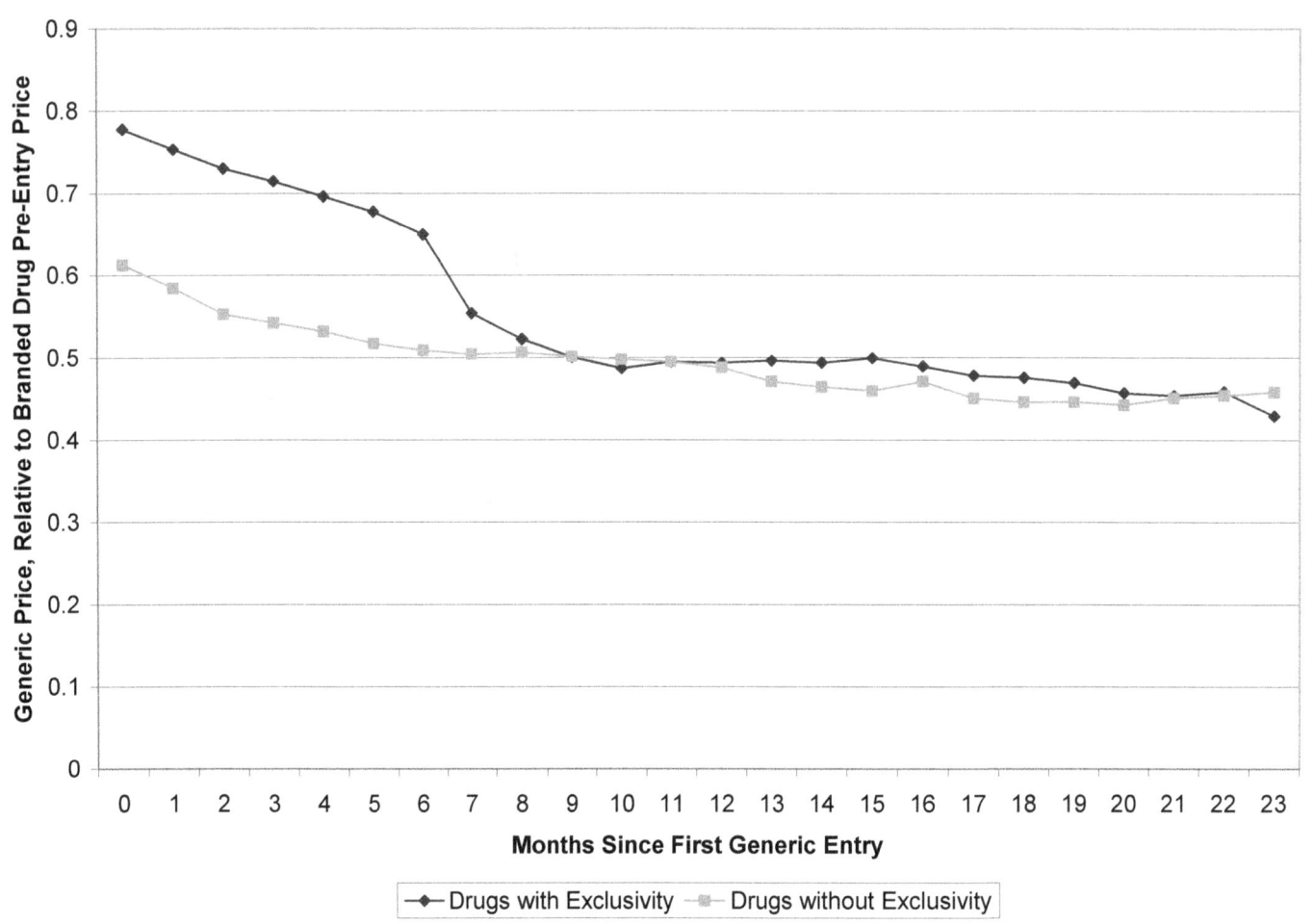

Notes: Branded drug price measured in the quarter prior to first generic entry.

www.ingramcontent.com/pod-product-compliance
Lightning Source LLC
Chambersburg PA
CBHW080758290526
45790CB00008B/3498